AF323698

Air Fryer Seafood and Vegetarian Recipes

A Collection of Delicious Recipes with no Meat for Preparing Healthy Meals With your Air Fryer

By Donna Thomson

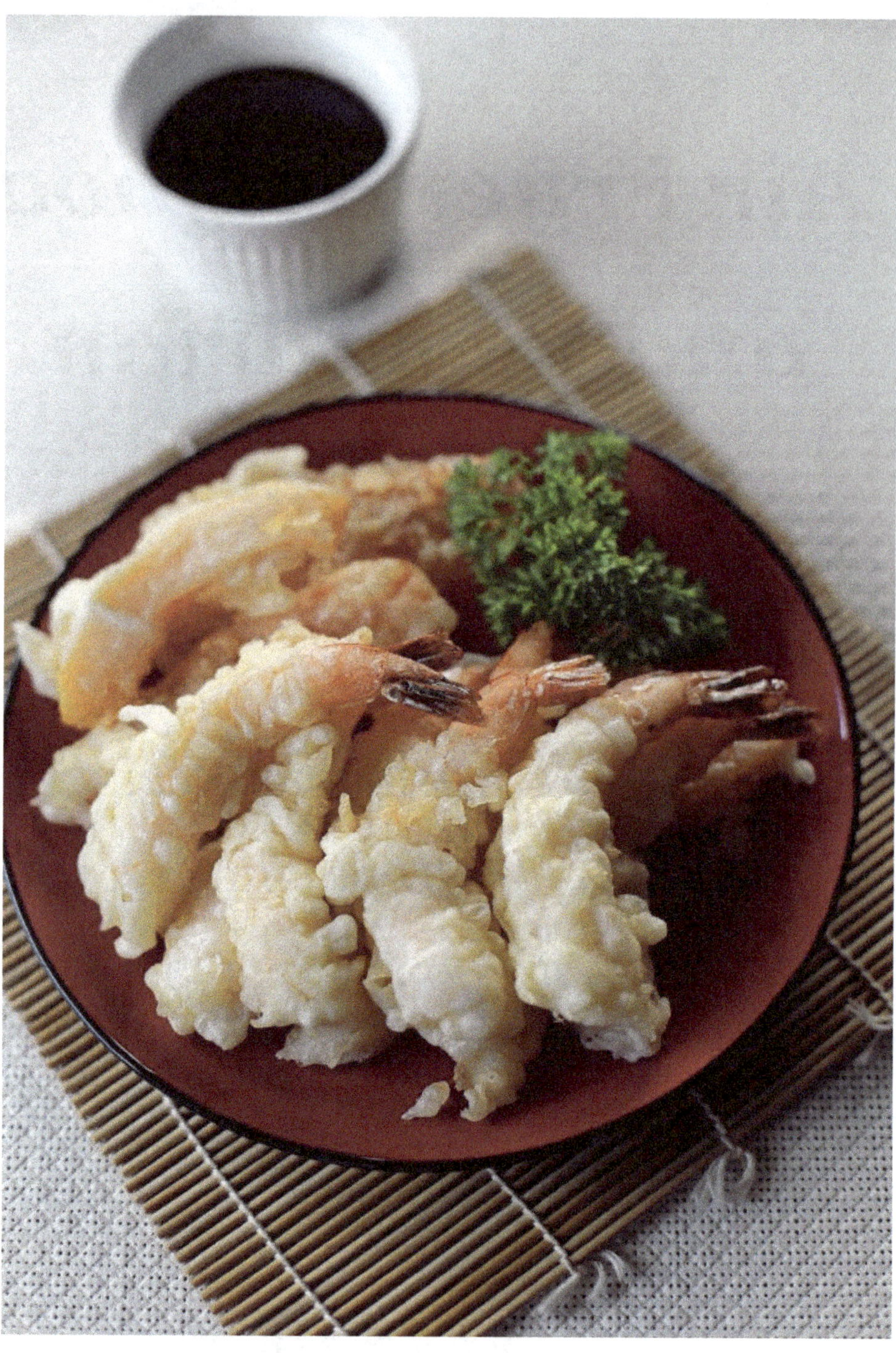

licensed professional before attempting any techniques outlined in this book.

By reading this document, the reader agrees that under no circumstances is the author responsible for any losses, direct or indirect, which are incurred as a result of the use of information contained within this document, including, but not limited to, — errors, omissions, or inaccuracies.

Table of Contents

SEAFOOD RECIPES.. 11

Kashmiri Chili Powder 'n Garlic Shrimp BBQ..................... 12

Lemony-Parsley Linguine with Grilled Tuna 15

Lemon-Basil on Cod Filet 17

Lemon-Garlic on Buttered Shrimp Fry 19

Lemon-Paprika Salmon Filet..21

Lemon-Pepper Red Mullet Fry 23

Lemony Grilled Halibut 'n Tomatoes 24

Lemony Tuna-Parsley Patties 27

Lemony-Sage on Grilled Swordfish 29

Lime 'n Chat masala Rubbed Snapper...............................31

Lime, Oil 'n Leeks on Grilled Swordfish 33

Lobster-Spinach Lasagna Recipe from Maine.................... 34

Mango Salsa on Fish Tacos 36

Miso Sauce Over Grilled Salmon 38

Old Bay 'n Dijon Seasoned Crab Cakes........................... 40

Orange Roughie with Caesar & Cheese Dressing 42

Oregano & Cumin Flavored Salmon Grill.......................... 43

Outrageous Crispy Fried Salmon Skin........................... 46

Pesto Basted Shrimp about the Grill 48

Pesto Sauce Over Fish Filet.. 49

Pina Colada Sauce Over Coconut Shrimps 51

Quick 'n Easy Tuna-Mac Casserole.................................... 53

Salad Nicosia With Peppery Halibut 55

Salmon Topped with Creamy Avocado-Cashew Sauce 57

Salted Tequila 'n Lime Shrimp 60

Savory Bacalao Tapas Recipe From Portugal 62

Shrimp, Mushroom 'n Rice Casserole 65

Soy-Orange Flavored Squid 67

Spiced Coco-Lime Skewered Shrimp.................................. 69

Sweet Honey-Hoisin Glazed Salmon 71

Sweet-Chili Sauce Dip 'n Shrimp Rolls.............................. 73

Tartar Sauce 'n Crispy Cod Nuggets 75

Tomato 'n Onion Stuffed Grilled Squid 78

Tortilla-Crusted with Lemon Filets 80

Turmeric Spiced Salmon with Soy Sauce 82

Very Easy Lime-Garlic Shrimps... 84

VEGETARIAN RECIPES... 86

Almond Flour Battered 'n Crisped Onion Rings 87

Almond Flour Battered Wings... 89

Baby Corn in Chili-Turmeric Spice 91

Baked Cheesy Eggplant with Marinara 93

Baked Polenta with Chili-Cheese 96

Baked Portobello, Pasta 'n Cheese 98

Baked Potato Topped with Cream cheese 'n Olives 100

Baked Zucchini Recipe From Mexico 102

Banana Pepper Stuffed with Tofu 'n Spices 104

Bell Pepper-Corn Wrapped in Tortilla 106

Black Bean Burger with Garlic-Chipotle 108

SEAFOOD RECIPES

Kashmiri Chili Powder 'n Garlic Shrimp BBQ

Servings per Recipe: 4

Cooking Time: 10

Ingredients:

- 1 fresh red Chile (like Fresno), seeds removed, finely grated
- 1 tablespoon coarsely ground pepper /15g
- 1 tablespoon fresh lime juice /15ml
- 1-pound large shrimp, peeled, deveined /450g
- 2 tablespoons vegetable oil, plus more for the grill /30ml
- 3 garlic cloves, finely grated
- Kosher salt
- Lime wedges and Kashmiri chili powder or paprika (for serving)

Instructions:

1) In a large bowl, combine oil, lime juice, pepper, garlic, and Chile. Add the shrimp season with salt and let it marinate for 10 minutes.
2) Thread shrimp into steel skewers.
3) Place on skewer rack in the air fryer.
4) Cook for 5 minutes at 3900 F or 199°C .
5) Dress in chili powder, lime wedges and serve.

Nutrition Information:

- Calories per Serving: 144
- Carbs: 2.2g
- Protein: 15.6g
- Fat: 8.0g

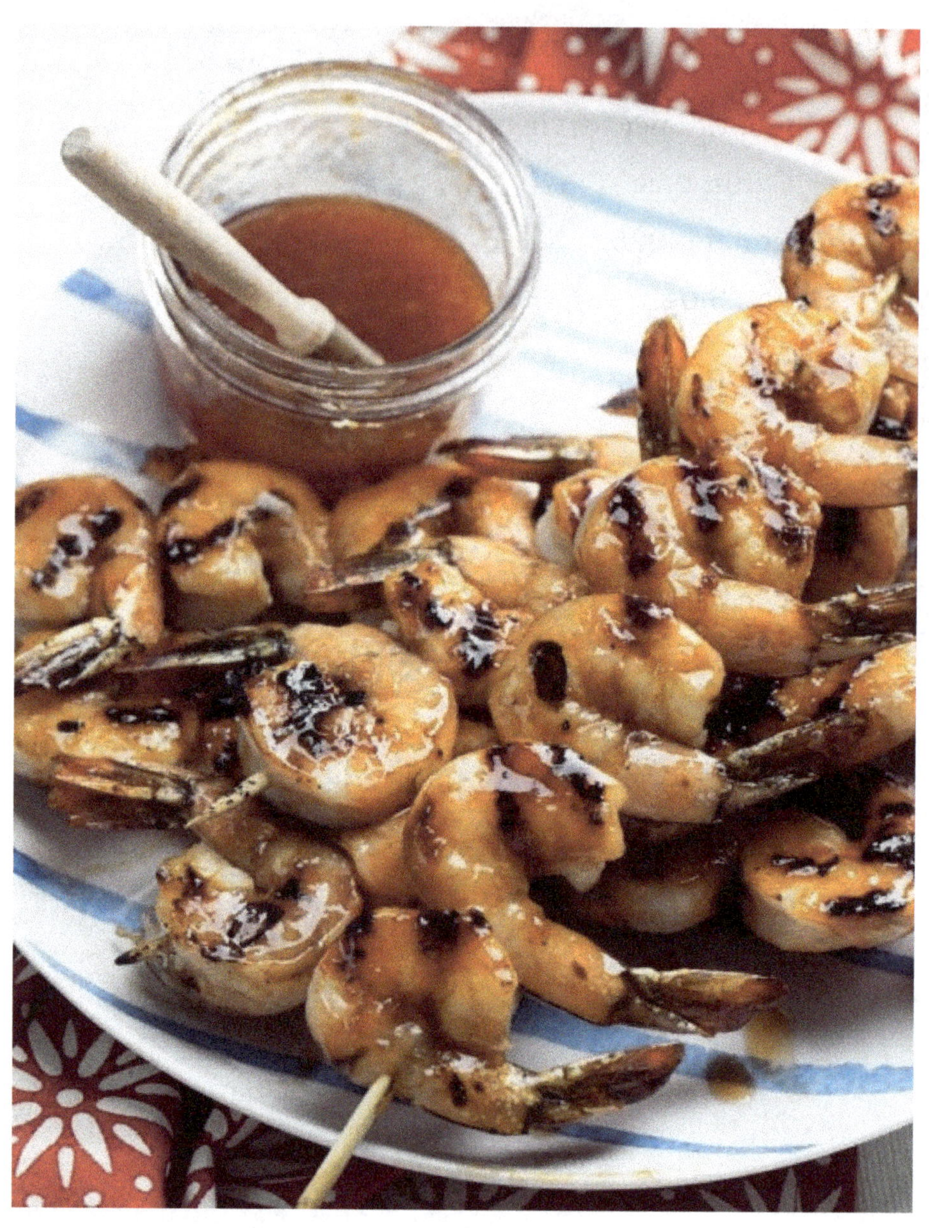

Lemony-Parsley Linguine with Grilled Tuna

Servings per Recipe: 2

Cooking Time: 20 Minutes

Ingredients:

- 1 tablespoon capers, chopped /15g
- 1 tablespoon organic olive oil /15ml
- 12 ounces linguine, cooked based on package Instructions /360g
- 1-pound fresh tuna fillets /450g
- 2 cups parsley leaves, chopped /260g
- Juice from 1 lemon
- Salt and pepper to taste

Instructions:

1) Preheat the air fryer to 3900 F or 199°C .
2) Place the grill pan in the air fryer.
3) Season both sides of the tuna with salt and pepper. polish with oil.
4) Grill for 20 minutes.
5) Shred cooked tuna into pieces using a fork and serve with cooked linguine. Sprinkle parsley and capers. Season with salt and pepper to taste and sprinkle with freshly squeezed lemon juice.

Nutrition information:

- Calories per serving: 520
- Carbs: 60.6g
- Protein: 47.7g
- Fat: 9.6g

Lemon-Basil on Cod Filet

Servings per Recipe: 4

Cooking Time: 15

Ingredients:

- ¼ cup essential olive oil /62.5ML
- 4 cod fillets
- A lot of basil, torn
- Juice from 1 lemon, freshly squeezed
- Salt and pepper to taste

Instructions:

1) Warm air fryer for 5 minutes.
2) Season the cod fillets with salt and pepper to taste. Place in a sparingly greased baking pan.
3) Mix the remainder of the ingredients inside a bowl and stir to combine well. Pour over the fish.
4) Cook for 15 minutes at 330° F or 166°C .
5) Serve and enjoy.

Nutrition information:

- Calories per serving: 235
- Cars: 1.9g
- Protein: 14.3g
- Fat: 18.9g

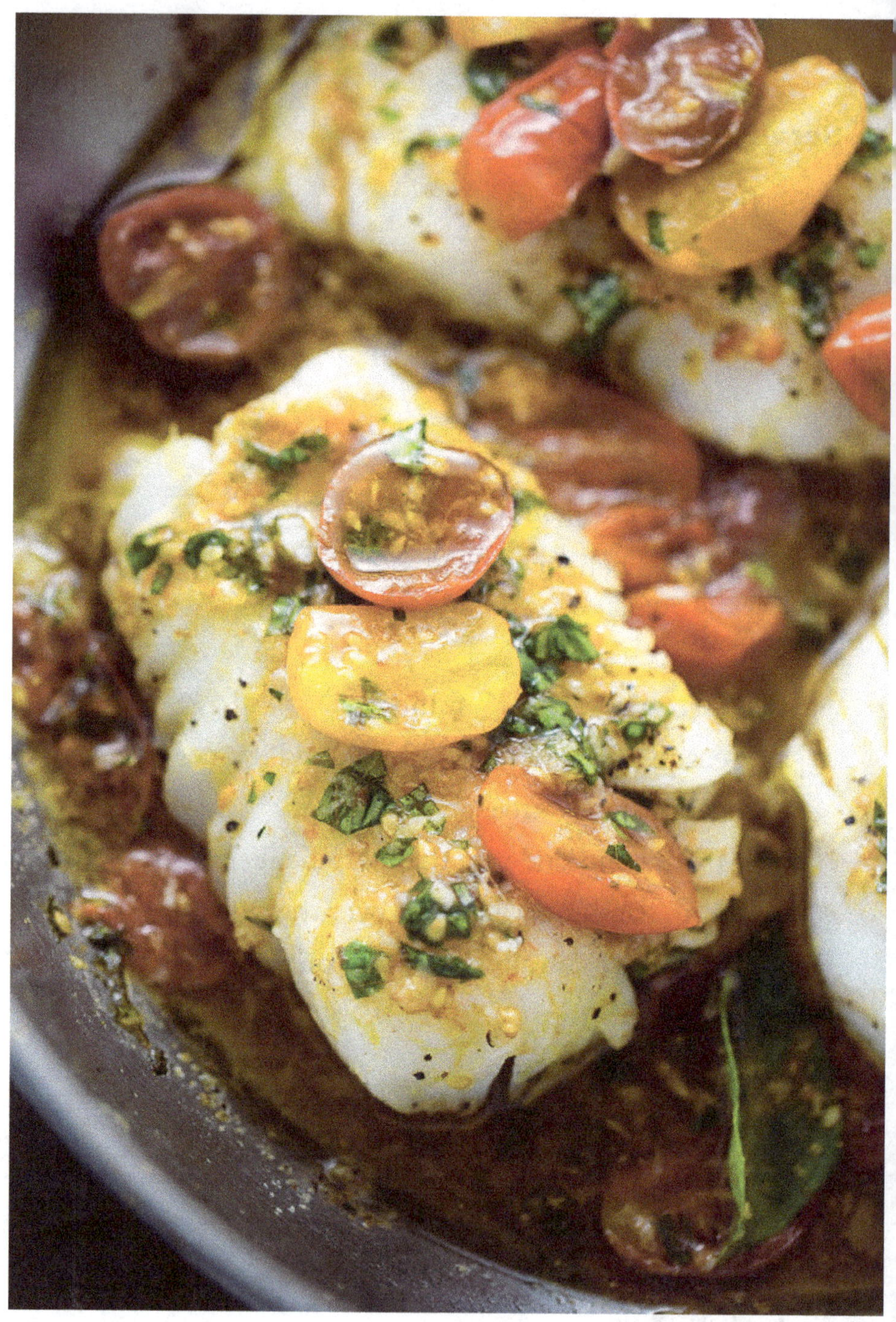

Lemon-Garlic on Buttered Shrimp Fry

Servings per Recipe: 4

Cooking Time: 15

Ingredients:

- 1 tablespoon chopped chives or 1 teaspoon dried chives /15G OR /5G
- 1 tablespoon freshly squeezed lemon juice /15ML
- 1tablespoon minced basil leaves plus more for sprinkling or 1 teaspoon dried basil /15G
- 1 tablespoon minced garlic /15G
- 1-lb defrosted shrimp (21-25 count) /450G
- 2 tablespoons chicken stock (or white wine) /30ML
- 2 teaspoons red pepper flakes /10G
- 4 tablespoons butter /60G

Instructions

1) Lightly grease the baking dish with cooking spray using any oil of your choice. Melt the butter for two minutes at 330°F or 166°C. Add red pepper flakes and garlic. Cook for 3 minutes.
2) Add remaining ingredients to a pan and Stir well to coat completely.
3) Cook for 5 minutes at 330°F or 166°C . Stir and allow it to cook for another 5 minutes.

4) Serve and enjoy

Nutrition Information:

- Calories per Serving: 213
- Carbs: 1.0g
- Protein: 23.0g
- Fat: 13.0g

Lemon-Paprika Salmon Filet

Servings per Recipe: 2

Cooking Time: 15

Ingredients:

- 1 tablespoon butter, melted /15ML
- 1 tablespoon minced fresh thyme or 1 teaspoon dried thyme /15G
- 1 teaspoon grated lemon zest /5G
- 1/2 teaspoon salt /2.5G
- 1/4 teaspoon lemon-pepper seasoning /1.25G
- 1/4 teaspoon paprika /1.25
- 1-1/2 cups soft bread crumbs /195G
- 2 garlic cloves, minced
- 2 salmon fillets (6 ounces or /180G each)
- 2 tablespoons minced fresh parsley /30G

Instructions

1) Add bread crumbs, fresh parsley thyme, garlic, lemon zest, salt, lemon-pepper seasoning, and paprika in a medium-sized bowl. Stir to combine well.
2) Lightly grease the baking dish with oil. Add salmon filet with the skin facing down. Evenly sprinkle bread crumbs on top of the salmon.

3) Cook for 10 minutes at 390°F or 199°C . Allow to sit for 5 minutes.

4) Serve and Enjoy

Nutrition Information:

- Calories per Serving: 331
- Carbs: 9.0g
- Protein: 31.0g
- Fat: 19.0g

Lemon-Pepper Red Mullet Fry

Servings per Recipe: 4

Cooking Time: 15

Ingredients:

- 1 tablespoon olive oil /15ML
- 4 whole red mullets, gutted and scales removed
- Juice from 1 lemon
- Salt and pepper to taste

Instructions:

1) Preheat the air fryer to 390° F or 199°C .
2) Place the grill pan in the air fryer.
3) Season the red mullet with salt, pepper, and lemon juice.
4) Brush with extra virgin olive oil.
5) Grill for 15 minutes per batch.

Nutrition information:

- Calories per serving: 152
- Carbs: 0.9g
- Protein: 23.1g
- Fat: 6.2g

Lemony Grilled Halibut 'n Tomatoes

Servings per Recipe: 4

Cooking Time: 15

Ingredients:

- ½ cup hearts of palm, rinse and drained /65G
- 1 cup cherry tomatoes /130
- 2 tablespoons oil /30ML
- 4 halibut fillets
- Juice from 1 lemon
- Salt and pepper to taste

Instructions:

1) Preheat the air fryer to 390° F or 199°C .
2) Place the grill pan in the air fryer.
3) Season the halibut fillets with lemon juice, salt and pepper to taste. Brush with your preferred oil.
4) Place the fish in the grill pan.
5) Arrange the hearts of palms and cherry tomatoes on the side and sprinkle with more salt and pepper.
6) Allow cooking for 15 minutes.

Nutrition information:

- Calories per serving: 208
- Carbs: 7g

- Protein: 21 g
- Fat: 11g

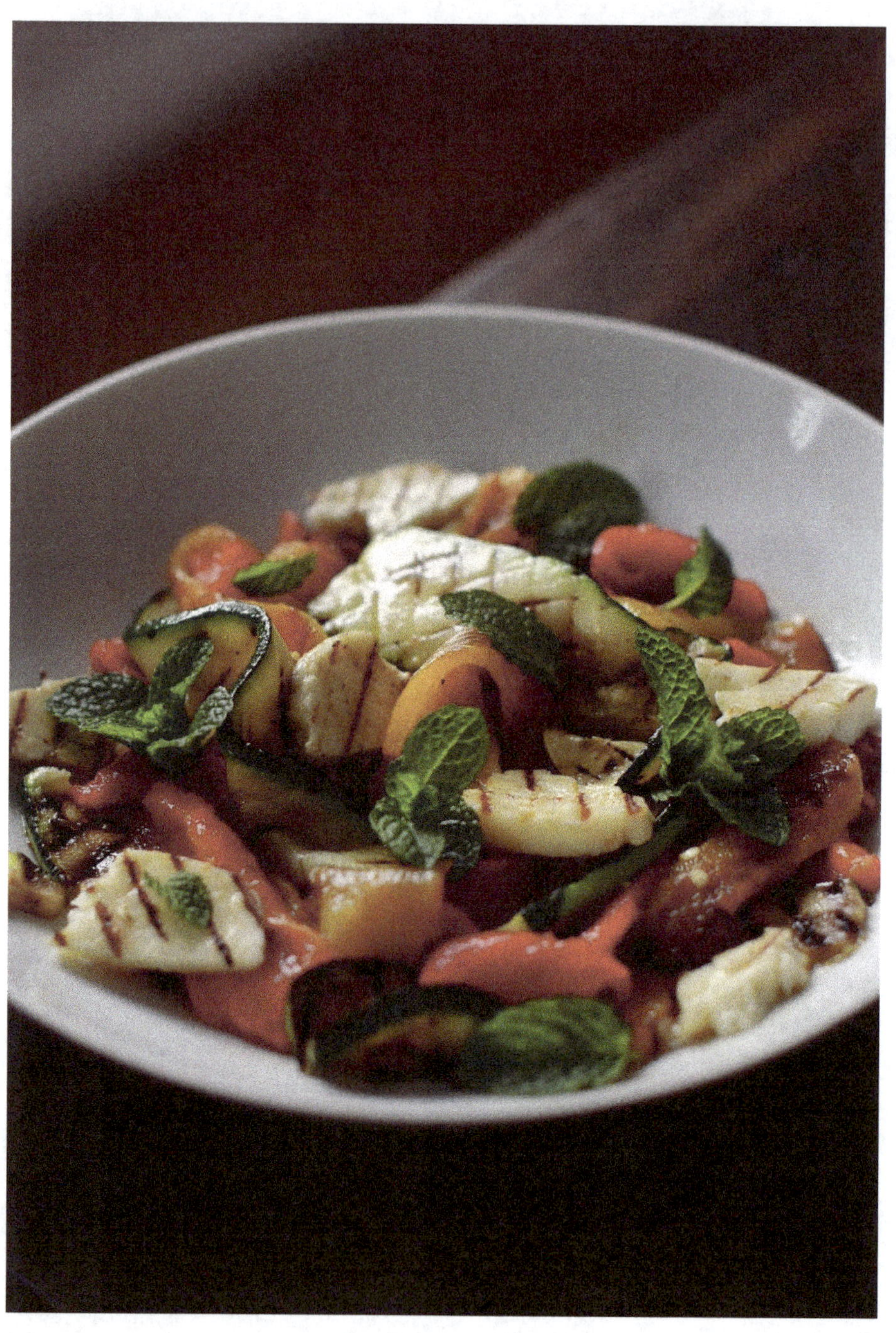

Lemony Tuna-Parsley Patties

Servings per Recipe: 4

Cooking Time: 10 Minutes

Ingredients

- ½ cup panko bread crumbs /65G
- 1 egg, beaten
- 1 tablespoon freshly squeezed lemon juice /15ML
- 2 cans of tuna in brine
- 2 tablespoons chopped parsley /30G
- 2 teaspoons Dijon mustard /30G
- 3 tablespoons extra virgin olive oil /45ML
- A drizzle of Tabasco sauce

Instructions:

1) Remove the liquid from the canned tuna and set it in the bowl.
2) Shred the tuna in a bowl and season with mustard, bread crumbs, fresh lemon juice, and parsley.
3) Add the egg and Tabasco sauce to the mix. Stir until well combined.
4) Form shaped lumps using your hands and place them inside the fried setting for about 120 minutes.
5) Preheat mid-air fryer to 390° F or 199°C .
6) Place the grill pan in the air fryer.

7) Brush all sides of the patties with essential olive oil, place in the grill pan.

8) Cook for 10 minutes. Turn over the patties after 5 minutes for even browning.

Nutrition information:

- Calories per serving: 209
- Carbs: 2.9g
- Protein: 18.8g
- Fat: 13.5g

Lemony-Sage on Grilled Swordfish

Servings per Recipe: 2

Cooking Time: 16 minutes

Ingredients:

- ½ lemon, sliced thinly in rounds
- 1 tbsp fresh lemon juice /15ML
- 1 tsp parsley /5G
- 1 zucchini, peeled after which thinly sliced in lengths
- 1/2-pound swordfish, sliced into 2-inch chunks /225G
- 2 tbsp extra virgin olive oil /30ML
- 6-8 sage leaves
- salt and pepper to taste

Instructions:

1) Mix freshly squeezed lemon juice, parsley, and sliced swordfish in a shallow bowl. Stir well to coat and season with pepper and salt as you prefer. Marinate for about 10 minutes.

2) Place a zucchini over a flat surface. Add one part of fish and sage leaf in the middle, roll up zucchini and then thread on a skewer. Repeat the process until all ingredients have been exhausted.

3) Brush with oil and place on a skewer rack in the air fryer.

4) For 8 minutes, cook at 390° F or 199°C . Cook in batches preferably.

5) Serve and enjoy with fresh lemon slices.

Nutrition Information:

- Calories per Serving: 297
- Carbs: 3.7g
- Protein: 22.8g
- Fat: 21.2g

Lime 'n Chat masala Rubbed Snapper

Servings per Recipe: 2

Cooking Time: 25 minutes

Ingredients:

- 1/3 cup chat masala /43G
- 1-1/2 pounds whole fish, cut by 50 per cent /675G
- 2 tablespoons organic olive oil /30ML
- 3 tablespoons fresh lime juice /45ML
- Salt to taste

Instructions:

1) Preheat mid-air fryer to 390° F or 199°C .
2) Place the grill pan in the air fryer.
3) Place fish on a flat surface and season the fish with salt, chat masala and lime juice.
4) Brush with oil
5) Place the fish in the air fryer's basket lined with foil.
6) Cook for 25 minutes. Turn over halfway through cooking time.

Nutrition information:

- Calories per serving:308
- Carbs: 0.7g
- Protein: 35.2g

- Fat: 17.4g

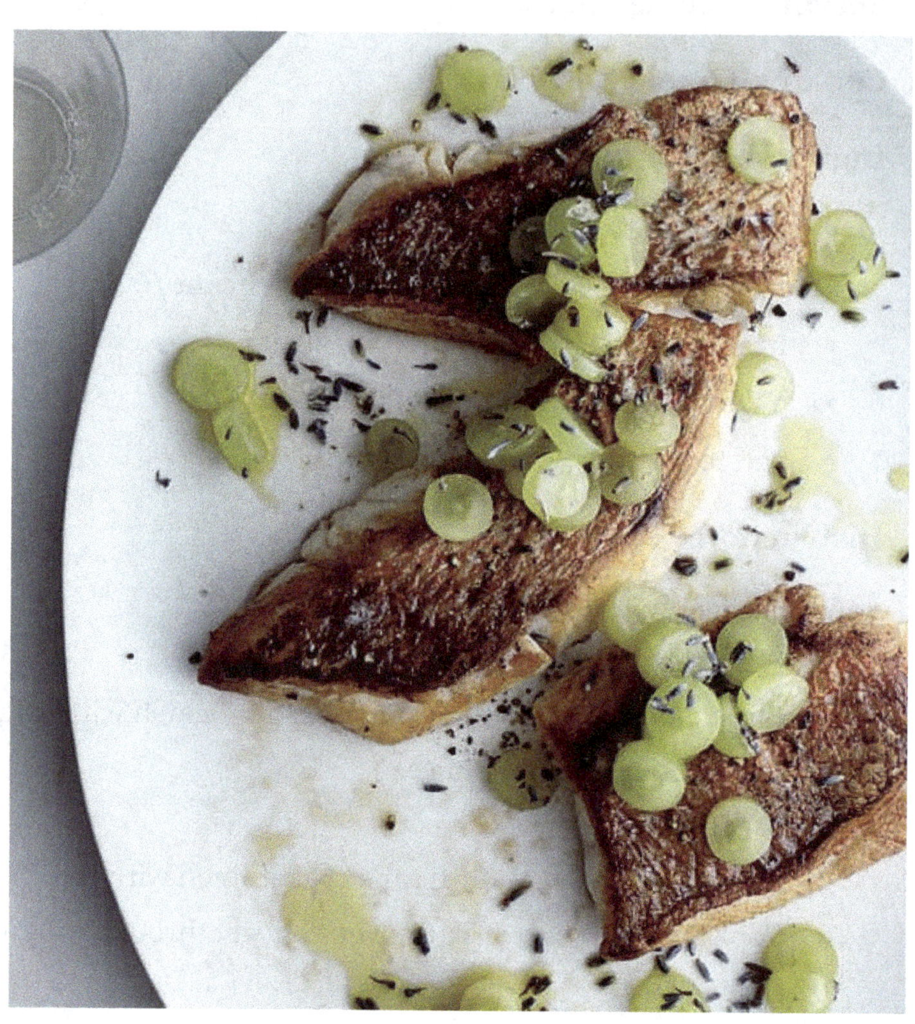

Lime, Oil 'n Leeks on Grilled Swordfish

Servings per Recipe: 4

Cooking Time: 20 Minutes

Ingredients:

- 2 tablespoons olive oil /30ML
- 3 tablespoons lime juice /45ML
- 4 medium leeks, cut into an inch long
- 4 swordfish steaks
- Salt and pepper to taste

Instructions:

1) Preheat air fryer to 390° F or 199°C .
2) Place the grill pan in the air fryer.
3) Season the swordfish with salt, pepper and lime juice.
4) Brush the fish with extra virgin olive oil
5) Place fish fillets in a grill pan and garnish with leeks.
6) Grill for 20 minutes.

Nutrition information:

- Calories per serving: 611
- Carbs: 14.6g
- Protein: 48g
- Fat: 40g

Lobster-Spinach Lasagna Recipe from Maine

Servings per Recipe: 6

Cooking Time: 50 minutes

Ingredients:

- 1 (16 ounces or 480G) jar Alfredo pasta sauce
- 1 cup shredded Cheddar cheese /130G
- 1 egg
- 1 pound cooked and cubed lobster meat /450G
- 1 tablespoon chopped fresh parsley /15G
- 1/2 (15 ounces or 450G) container ricotta cheese
- 1/2 cup grated Parmesan cheese /65G
- 1/2 cup shredded mozzarella cheese /65G
- 1/2 medium onion, minced
- 1/2 teaspoon freshly ground black pepper /2.5G
- 1-1/2 teaspoons minced garlic /7.5G
- 5-ounce package baby spinach leaves /150G
- 8 no-boil lasagna noodles

Instructions:

1) Mix 50% of Parmesan, half mozzarella, 50% of cheddar, egg, and ricotta cheese in a medium-sized bowl. Sprinkle pepper, parsley, garlic, and onion.

2) Lightly grease baking pan of air fryer with cooking spray using any oil of your choice.

3) Spread ½ of the Alfredo sauce in the baking pan. Sprinkle a single layer of lasagna noodles on it, also place 1/3 of lobster meat, 1/3 of ricotta cheese mixture, 1/3 of spinach. Repeat the layering process until all ingredients are exhausted.

4) Sprinkle remaining cheese on top. Shake pan for ingredients to set and for air bubbles to burst. Cover pan with foil.

5) Cook at 360° F for 30 minutes or 183°C .

6) Remove foil and cook for an additional 10 minutes at the same temperature until tops are lightly brown and the middle is set.

7) Let it cool for 10 minutes.

8) Serve, eat and enjoy.

Nutrition Information:

- Calories per Serving: 558
- Carbs: 20.4g
- Protein: 36.8g
- Fat: 36.5g

Mango Salsa on Fish Tacos

Servings per Recipe: 4

Cooking Time: 10

Ingredients:

- ½ cup mango salsa of your choice /65G
- 1 cup corn kernels /130G
- 1 cup mixed greens /130G
- 1 red bell pepper, seeded and diced
- 1 yellow onion, peeled and diced
- 4 large burrito-size tortillas
- 4 pieces of fish fillets
- Juice from ½ lemon
- Salt and pepper to taste

Instructions:

1) Preheat the air fryer to 330° F or 166°C .
2) Season the fish with freshly squeezed lemon juice, salt and pepper to taste.
3) Place seasoned fish on the double layer rack.
4) Cook for 10 minutes.
5) Place tortillas over a flat surface, add fish fillet, onions, pepper, corn kernels, and mixed greens. This will make 4 tortilla wraps
6) Serve with mango salsa.

Nutrition information:

- Calories per serving: 378
- Carbs: 36g
- Protein: 26.8g
- Fat: 14g

Miso Sauce Over Grilled Salmon

Servings per Recipe: 4

Cooking Time: 16 minutes

Ingredients:

- 1 1/4 pounds skinless salmon fillets, thinly sliced /562.5G
- 1/4 cup yellow miso paste /62.5ML
- 2 tablespoons mirin (Japanese rice wine) /30ML
- 2 teaspoons dashi powder /10G
- 2 teaspoons superfine sugar /10G
- Amaranth leaves (optional), for everyone
- Shichimi togarashi, to serve

Instructions:

1) Add sugar, mirin, dashi powder, and miso in a bowl and mix well.
2) Thread salmon into skewers. Drizzle with miso glaze. Place on skewer rack in the air fryer. If needed, cook in batches.
3) For 8 minutes, cook on 360° F or 183°C . Halfway through cooking time, turnover and drizzle with more miso glaze.
4) Serve and enjoy

Nutrition Information:

- Calories per Serving: 281
- Carbs: 7.6g
- Protein: 39.8g
- Fat: 10.1g

Old Bay 'n Dijon Seasoned Crab Cakes

Servings per Recipe: 2

Cooking Time: 10 minutes

Ingredients:

- ¼ cup chopped green onion /32.5G
- ½ cup panko /65G
- 1 ½ teaspoon old bay seasoning /7.5G
- 1 teaspoon Dijon mustard /5G
- 1 teaspoon Worcestershire sauce /5ML
- 1-pound lump crab meat /450G
- 2 large eggs
- Salt and pepper to taste

Instructions:

1) Preheat the air fryer to 390° F or 199°C .
2) Place the grill pan in the mid-air fryer.
3) In a mixing bowl, combine and stir all Ingredients until properly combined.
4) Form small patties of crab cakes using your hands.
5) Place on the grill pan and cook for 10 Minutes.
6) For even browning flip the crab cakes halfway through cooking time.

Nutrition information:

- Calories per serving: 129
- Carbs: 4.3g
- Protein: 16.2g
- Fat: 5.1g

Orange Roughie with Caesar & Cheese Dressing

Servings per Recipe: 2

Cooking Time: 15

Ingredients:

- 2 orange roughie fillets (4 ounces or /120G each)
- 1/2 cups crushed butter-flavored crackers /65G
- 1/2 cup shredded cheddar cheese /65G
- 1/4 cup creamy Caesar salad dressing /32.5G

Instructions:

1) Sparingly grease the baking pan with oil. Add filet to the bottom of the pan. Sprinkle with dressing and crumbled crackers.
2) Cook for 10 minutes at 390 ° F or 199°C .
3) Sprinkle cheese and allow it to sit for 5 minutes.
4) Serve and enjoy

Nutrition Information:

- Calories per Serving: 341
- Carbs: 5.0g
- Protein: 32.6g
- Fat: 21.1g

Oregano & Cumin Flavored Salmon Grill

Servings per Recipe: 4

Cooking Time: 15

Ingredients:

- 1 1/2 pounds skinless salmon fillet (preferably wild), cut into 1" pieces /675G
- 1 teaspoon ground cumin /5G
- 1 teaspoon kosher salt /5G
- 1/4 teaspoon crushed red pepper flakes /1.25G
- 2 lemons, very thinly sliced into rounds
- 2 tablespoons chopped fresh oregano /30G
- 2 tablespoons essential olive oil /30ML
- 2 teaspoons sesame seeds /10G

Instructions:

1) In a small bowl, combine oregano, sesame seeds, cumin, salt, and pepper flakes. Stir well.
2) Thread salmon and folded lemon slices in a skewer. Brush with oil and dust with seasoning.
3) Place skewers on the air fryer skewer rack.
4) Allow cooking for 5 minutes at 360° F or 183°C . If needed, cook in batches.
5) Serve and enjoy

Nutrition Information:

- Calories per Serving: 313
- Carbs: 2.3g
- Protein: 34.3g
- Fat: 18.5g

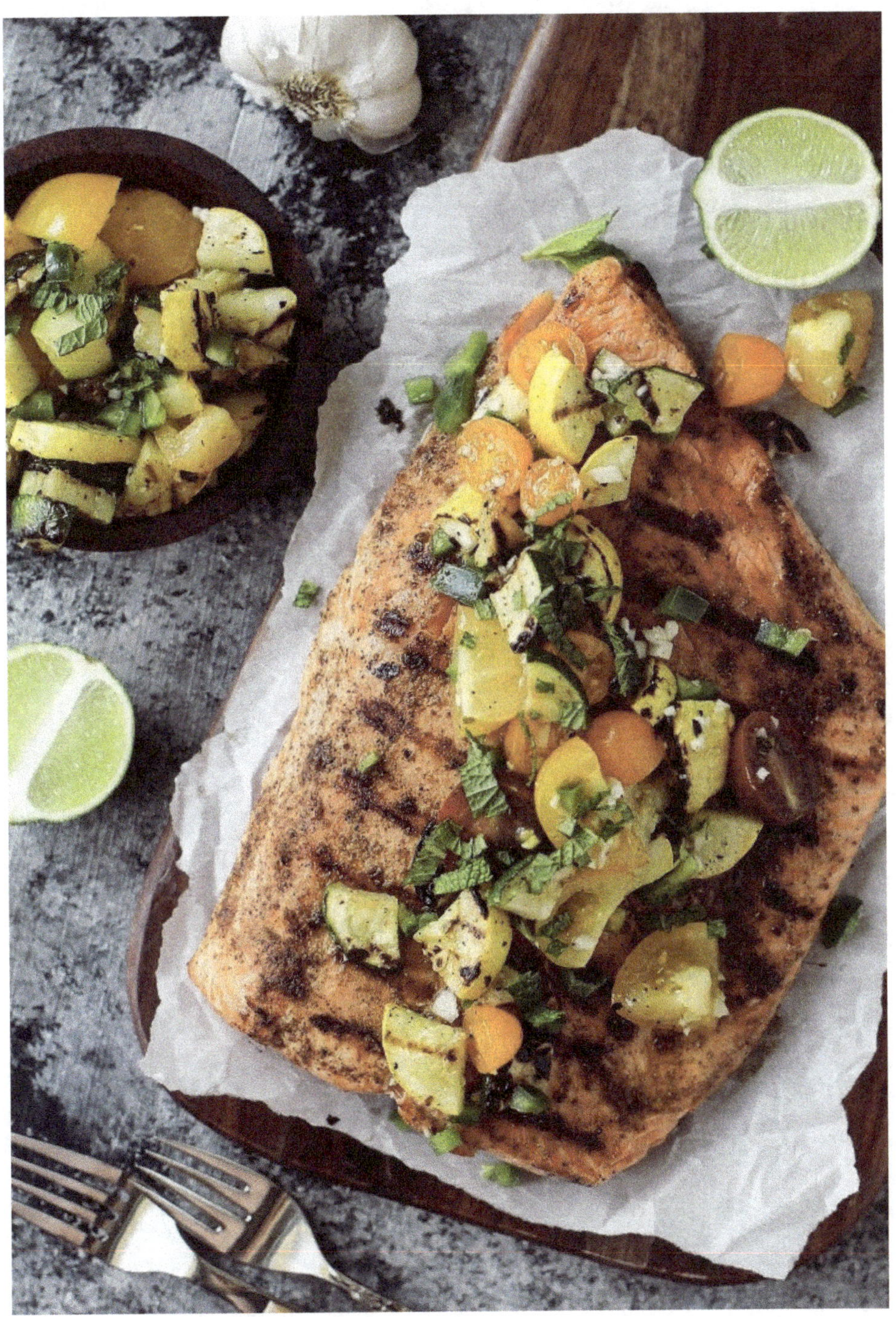

Outrageous Crispy Fried Salmon Skin

Serves: 4

Cooking Time: 10 minutes

Ingredients:

- ½ pound salmon skin patted dry /225G
- 4 tablespoons coconut oil /60ML
- Salt and pepper to taste

Instructions:

1) Preheat the air fryer for 5 minutes.
2) In a large mixing bowl, combine all ingredients and mix well.
3) Place inside fryer basket.
4) At 400° For 205°C cook for 10 minutes.
5) Shake the air fryer's basket halfway through cooking time to evenly cook the skin.

Nutrition information:

- Calories per serving: 221
- Carbohydrates: 1.1g
- Protein: 15.2g
- Fat: 16.9g

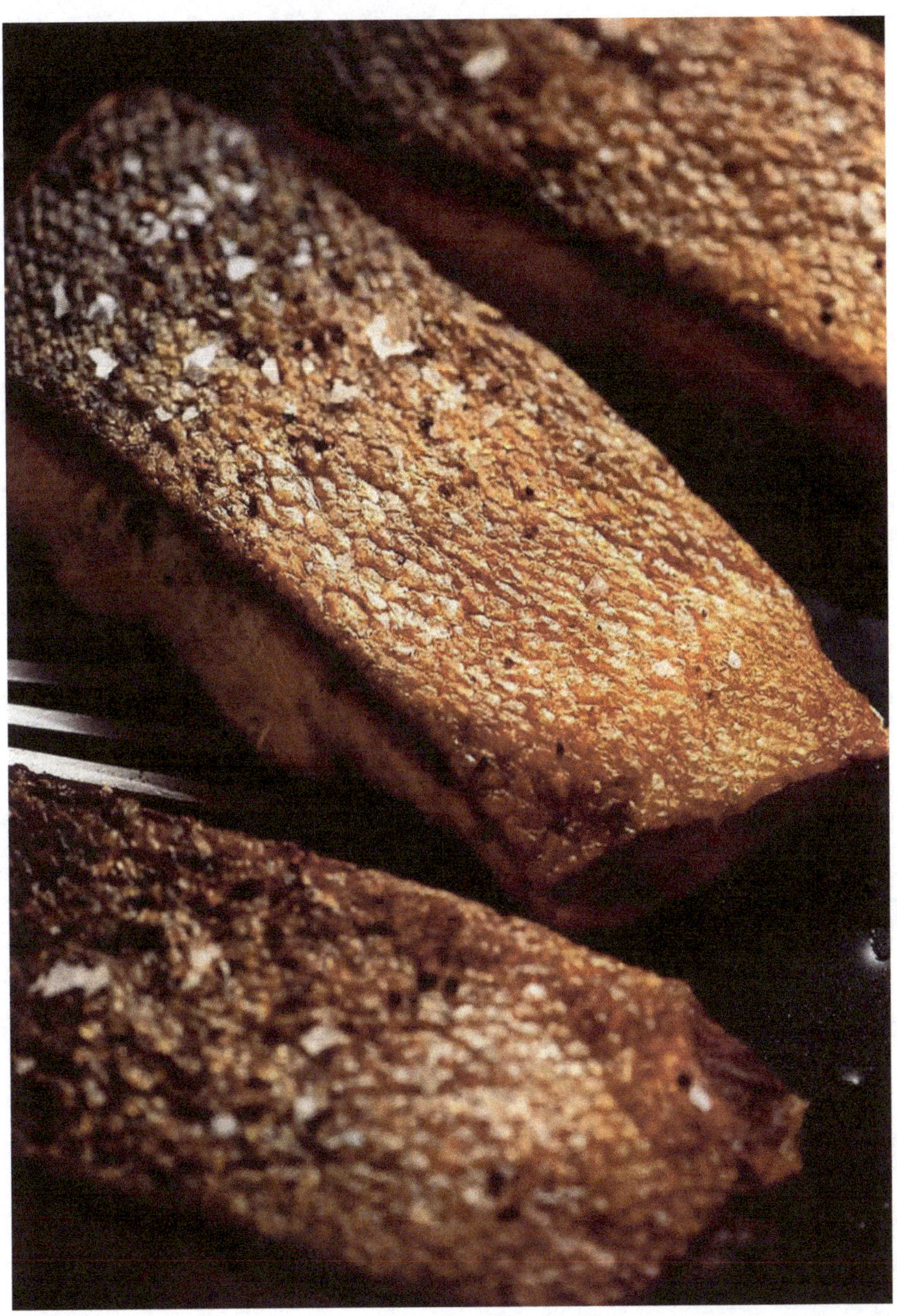

Pesto Basted Shrimp about the Grill

Servings per Recipe: 4

Cooking Time: 16 minutes

Ingredients:

- 1 cup pesto /130G
- 1/4 cup chopped fresh basil /32.5G
- 1-lb extra-large shrimp, peeled and deveined /450G
- bamboo skewers, soaked in water
- Extra-virgin extra virgin olive oil, for drizzling
- Freshly ground black pepper

Instructions:

1) Thread shrimp into skewers and set on skewer rack. Shower with oil, season with pepper and salt to taste.
2) At 360° F or 183°C cook for 8 minutes. Turnover halfway through cooking time while sprinkling the shrimps with pesto.
3) Dress with fresh basil, serve and enjoy.

Nutrition Information:

- Calories per Serving: 544
- Carbs: 9.6g
- Protein: 7.0g
- Fat: 53.0

Pesto Sauce Over Fish Filet

Serves: 3

Cooking Time: 20 minutes

Ingredients:

- 1 bunch of fresh basil
- 1 cup organic olive oil /250ML
- 1 tablespoon parmesan cheese, grated /15G
- 2 cloves of garlic,
- 2 tablespoons pine nuts /30G
- 3 white fish fillets
- Salt and pepper to taste

Instructions:

1) Get a mixing bowl, place all ingredients in it except the fish fillets. Mix properly
2) Beat until smooth.
3) Place the fish in a baking pan and pour in the pesto sauce.
4) Place in the air fryer and cook for 20 minutes at 400° F or 205°C .

Nutrition information:

- Calories per serving: 191
- Carbohydrates: 9.5g
- Protein: 8.2g

- Fat: 13.3g

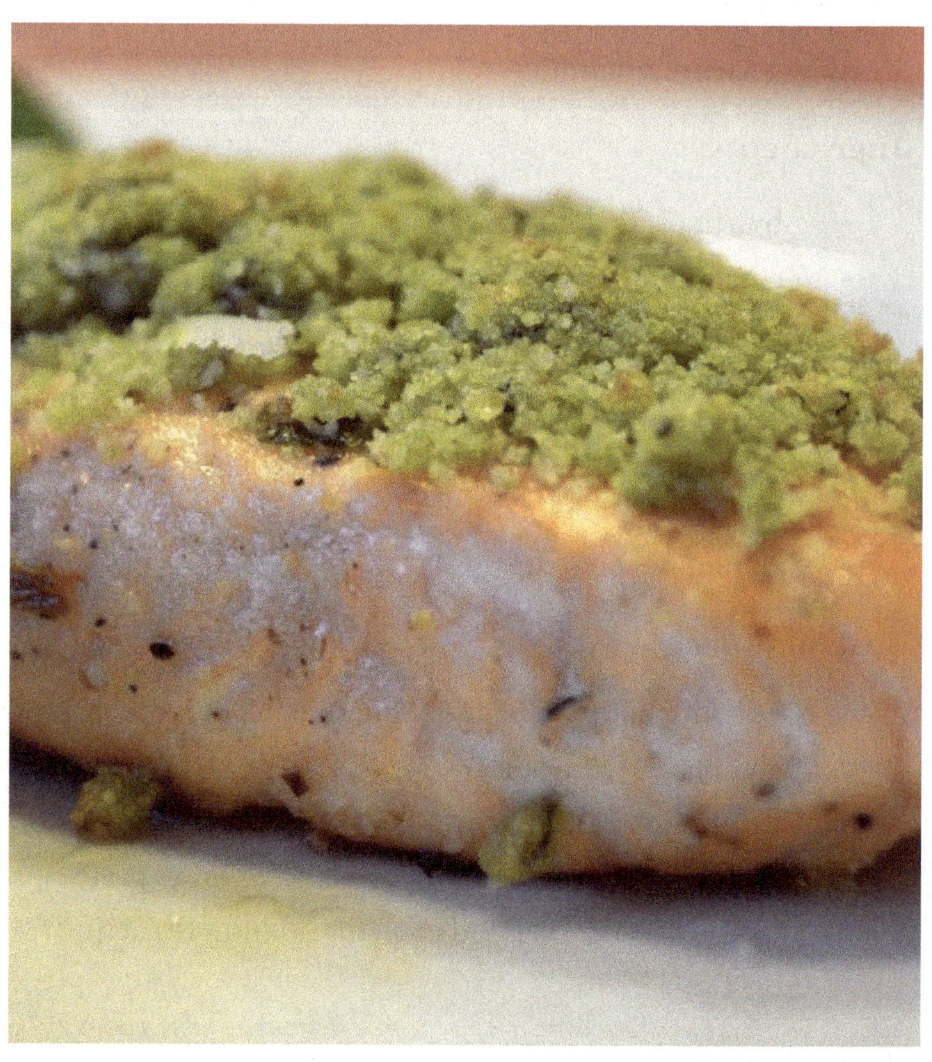

Pina Colada Sauce Over Coconut Shrimps

Servings per Recipe: 4

Cooking Time: 6 minutes

Ingredients:

- ¼ cup pineapple chunks, drained /32.5G
- ½ cup cornstarch /65G
- ¾ cups panko bread crumbs /88G
- 1 ½ pounds jumbo shrimps, peeled and deveined /675G
- 1 cup shredded coconut flakes /130G
- 1/3 cup light coconut milk /83ML
- 1/3 cup non-fat Greek yogurt /43G
- 2 tablespoons honey /30ML
- 2/3 cup coconut milk /166ML
- Salt and pepper to taste
- Toasted coconut meat for garnish

Instructions:

1) Preheat air fryer to 390° F or 199°C .
2) In a large Ziploc bag, place the shrimps and cornstarch, shake excellently.

3) In a mixing bowl, add coconut milk and honey. Stir well to combine. Set aside.
4) In another mixing bowl, mix the coconut flakes and bread crumbs. Set aside.
5) Dip the shrimps inside the milk mixture then dip inside the bread crumbs. Coat properly.
6) Place inside the double layer rack and cook for 6 minutes.
7) Meanwhile, combine other ingredients to make the dipping sauce.

Nutrition information:

- Calories per serving: 493
- Carbs: 21.4g
- Protein: 38.9g
- Fat: 27.9g

Quick 'n Easy Tuna-Mac Casserole

Servings per Recipe: 4

Cooking Time: 20 minutes

Ingredients:

- 1/2 (10.75 ounces or 322.5 ML) can condensed cream of chicken soup
- 1-1/2 cups cooked macaroni /195G
- 1/2 (5 ounces or 150G) can tuna, drained
- 1/2 cup shredded Cheddar cheese /65G
- 3/4 cup French fried onions /98G

Instructions:

1) Lightly grease the baking pan with oil.
2) Mix soup, tuna, and macaroni in a pan. Sprinkle cheese on top.
3) At 360° F or 183°C cook for 15 minutes. Bring out.
4) Sprinkle fried onions.
5) Cook for an additional 5 minutes.
6) Serve and enjoy.

Nutrition Information:

- Calories per Serving: 411
- Carbs: 37.1g
- Protein: 11.5g

- Fat: 28.5g

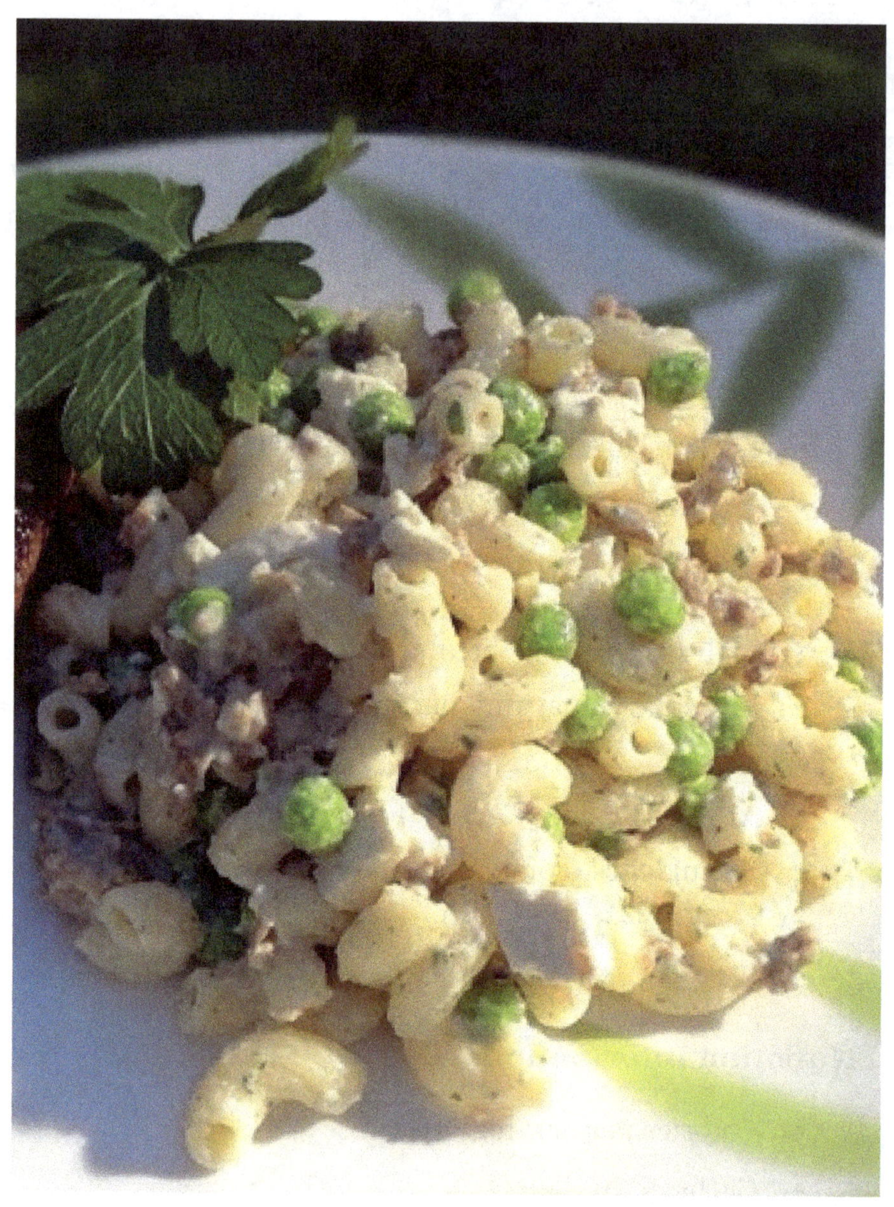

Salad Nicosia With Peppery Halibut

Servings per Recipe: 6

Cooking Time: 15

Ingredients:

- 1 ½ pounds halibut fillets /675G
- 1 cup cherry tomatoes, halved /130G
- 2 pounds mixed vegetables /900G
- 2 tablespoons extra virgin olive oil /30ML
- 4 cups torn lettuce leaves /520G
- 4 large hard-boiled eggs, peeled and sliced
- Salt and pepper to taste

Instructions:

1) Preheat mid-air fryer to 390 ° F or 199°C .
2) Place the grill pan in the air fryer.
3) Sprinkle the halibut with salt and pepper. Brush with oil.
4) Place on the grill.
5) Envelop the fish fillet with the mixed vegetables and cook for 15 minutes.
6) Prepare the salad by serving the fish fillet with grilled mixed vegetables, lettuce, cherry tomatoes, and hard-boiled eggs.

Nutrition information:

- Calories per serving: 312
- Carbs:16.8 g
- Protein: 19.8g
- Fat: 18.3g

Salmon Topped with Creamy Avocado-Cashew Sauce

Serves: 2

Cooking Time: 15 minutes

Ingredients:

- ½ clove of garlic
- ½ pound salmon fillet /225G
- 1 avocado, pitted and chopped
- 1 teaspoon organic olive oil /5ML
- 2 tablespoons cashew nuts, soaked in water for 10 minutes /30G
- Salt and pepper to taste

Instructions:

1) Warm up the air fryer for 5 minutes
2) Season the salmon fillets with salt, pepper, and essential olive oil.
3) Place in the air fryer and cook for 15 minutes at 400° F or 205°C .
4) Meanwhile, add all the remaining ingredients to a food processor. Season with salt and blend until smooth.
5) Serve the salmon fillet with creamy avocado sauce.

Nutrition information:

- Calories per serving: 417
- Carbohydrates: 13.7g
- Protein: 23.4g
- Fat: 29.8g

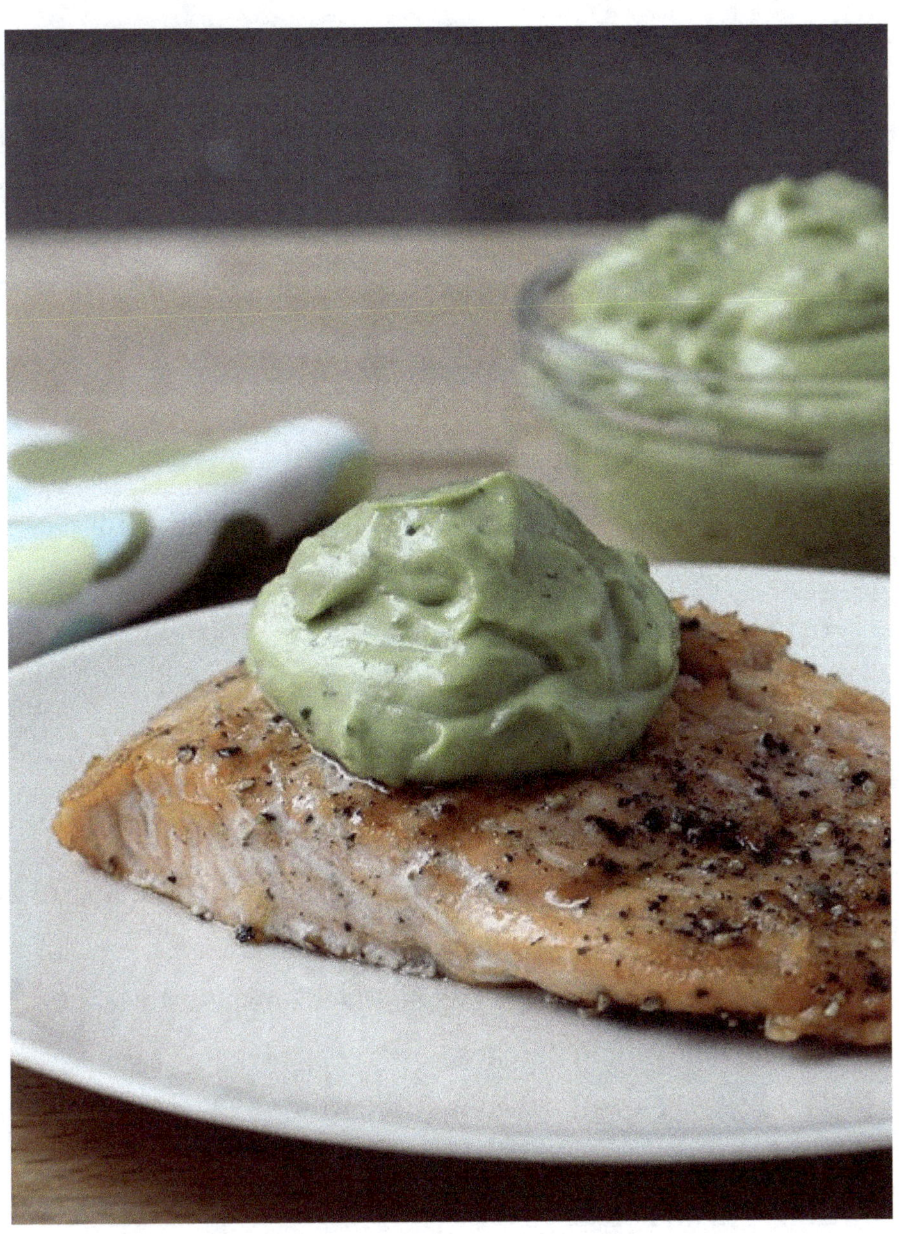

Salted Tequila 'n Lime Shrimp

Servings per Recipe: 3

Cooking Time: 16 minutes

Ingredients:

- 1 large lime, quartered
- 1 pinch garlic salt
- 1 pinch ground cumin
- 1/4 cup essential olive oil /62.5ML
- 1-pound large shrimp, peeled and deveined /450G
- 2 tablespoons lime juice /30ML
- 2 tablespoons tequila /30ML
- Ground black pepper to taste

Instructions:

1) Add pepper, cumin, salt, extra virgin olive oil, tequila and lime juice in a bowl. Dip the shrimp and marinate for at least one hour. Mixing once in a while.
2) Thread shrimps in skewers. Place on skewer rack. If needed cook in batches.
3) At 360° F or 183°C cook for 8 minutes. Turnover halfway through cooking time,
4) Serve and enjoy.

Nutrition Information:

- Calories per Serving: 222
- Carbs: 3.8g
- Protein: 18.8g
- Fat: 14.6g

Savory Bacalao Tapas Recipe From Portugal

Servings per Recipe: 4

Cooking Time: 26 minutes

Ingredients:

- 1 clove garlic, chopped, divided
- 1 yellow onions, thinly sliced
- 1/4 cup chopped fresh parsley, divided /32.5G
- 1/4 cup organic olive oil /62.5ML
- 1-pound codfish filet, chopped /450G
- 2 hard-cooked eggs, chopped
- 2 tablespoon butter /30G
- 2 Yukon Gold potatoes, peeled and diced
- 3/4 teaspoon red pepper flakes /3.75G
- 5 pitted black olives
- 5 pitted green olives
- freshly ground pepper to taste

Instructions:

1) Lightly grease the baking pan with oil. Add butter and melt at 360° F or 183°C . Add onions and cook for 6 minutes until transparent.

2) Add black pepper, red pepper flakes, 50% of parsley, garlic, organic olive oil, diced potatoes and chopped fish. At 360° F or 183°C cook for 10 minutes. Halfway through cooking time, stir well to mix.

3) At 390° F or 199°C cook for 10 minutes until the top is slightly brown.

4) Garnish with remaining parsley, eggs, black and green olives.

5) Serve and enjoy with chips.

Nutrition Information:

- Calories per Serving: 691
- Carbs: 25.2g
- Protein: 77.1g
- Fat: 31.3g

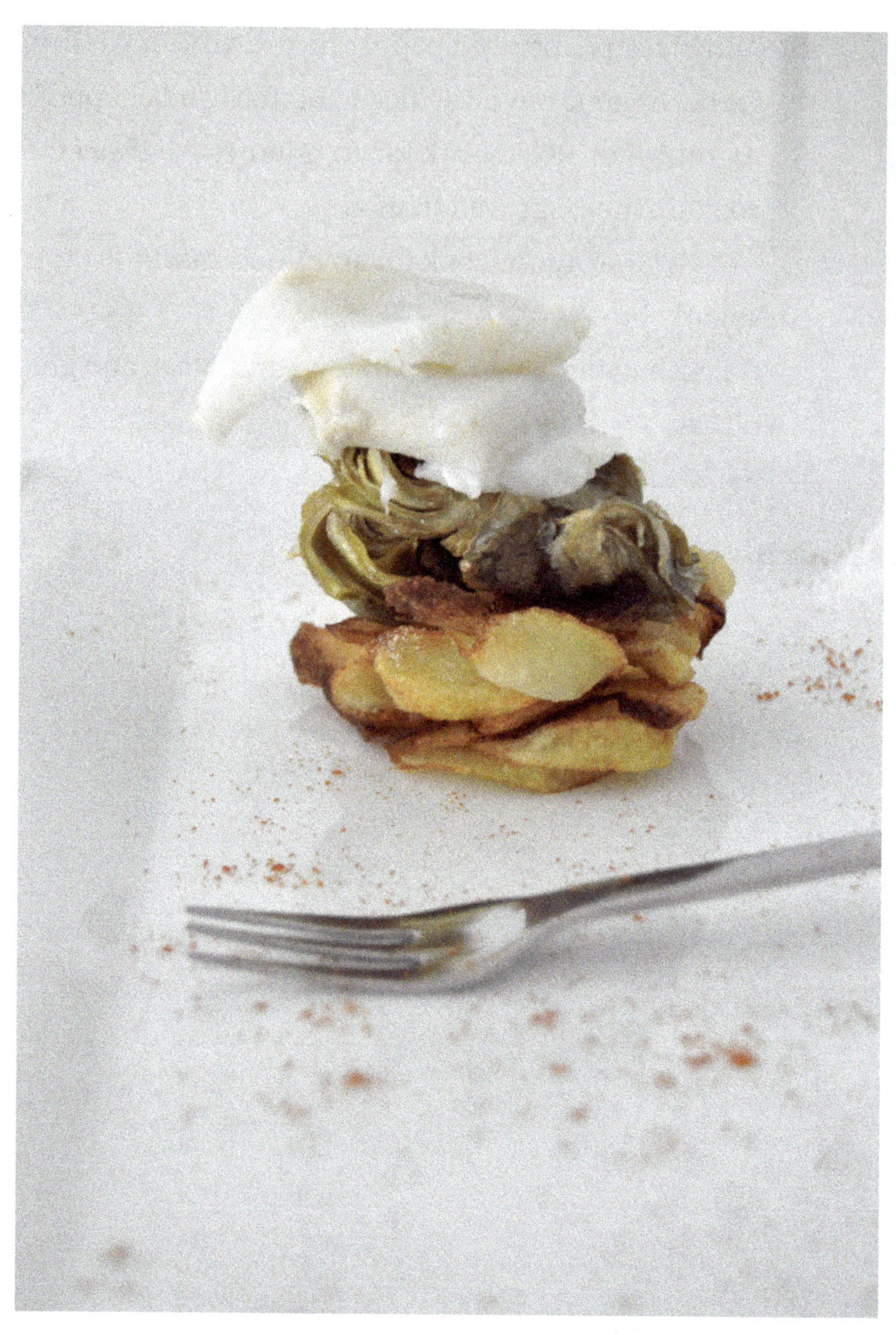

Shrimp, Mushroom 'n Rice Casserole

Servings per Recipe: 2

Cooking Time: 35 minutes

Ingredients:

- 1 tablespoon butter /15G
- 1/2 (10.75 ounces or 322.5ML) can condensed cream of shrimp soup
- 1/2 teaspoon vegetable oil /2.5ML
- 1/2-pound small shrimp, peeled and deveined /225G
- 1/2 (4 ounces or 120G) can sliced mushrooms, drained
- 1/2 (tall) container sour cream
- 1/3 cup shredded Cheddar cheese 43G
- 3/4 cup uncooked instant rice /98G
- 3/4 cup water /188ML

Instructions:

1) Lightly grease the baking pan with oil. Add rice, water, mushrooms, and butter. Cover with foil. For 20 minutes and cook at 360° F or 183°C .

2) Remove the foil cover, place in the shrimps, cover with foil and cook for additional 5 minutes.

3) Remove foil completely and stir in sour cream. Mix well and evenly spread rice.

4) Dress the top with cheese.

5) At 390° F or 199°C cook for 7 minutes until the top is lightly brown.

6) Serve and enjoy

Nutrition Information:

- Calories per Serving: 569
- Carbs: 38.5g
- Protein: 31.8g
- Fat: 31.9g

Soy-Orange Flavored Squid

Servings per Recipe: 4

Cooking Time: 10 minutes

Ingredients:

- ½ cup mirin /65G
- 1 cup soy sauce /250ML
- 1/3 cup yuzu or orange juice, freshly squeezed /83ML
- 2 cups water /500ML
- 2 pounds squid body, cut into rings /900G

Instructions:

1) Place all ingredients in a large Ziploc bag and place them in a fridge for some hours to allow the squid rings to marinate.
2) Preheat mid-air fryer to 390° F or 199°C .
3) Place the grill pan in the air fryer.
4) Grill the squid rings for 10 minutes.
5) While the squid is grilling, pour the marinade in a saucepan and allow it to simmer for 10 Minutes.
6) Drizzle the squid rings with all prepared sauce before serving.

Nutrition information:

- Calories per serving: 412

- Carbs: 4.1g
- Protein: 44.2g
- Fat: 24.3g

Spiced Coco-Lime Skewered Shrimp

Servings per Recipe: 6

Cooking Time: 12 minutes

Ingredients:

- 1 lime, zested and juiced
- 1/3 cup chopped fresh cilantro /43G
- 1/3 cup shredded coconut /43G
- 1/4 cup essential olive oil /62.5ML
- 1/4 cup soy sauce /62.5ML
- 1-pound uncooked medium shrimp, peeled and deveined /450G
- 2 garlic cloves
- 2 jalapeno peppers, seeded

Instructions:

1) Blend the soy sauce, extra virgin olive oil, coconut oil, cilantro, garlic, lime juice, lime zest, and jalapeno until smooth.
2) Mix shrimp and processed marinade in a bowl. Stir well to coat. Place in a fridge to marinate for 3 hours.
3) Thread shrimps in skewers. Place on skewer rack in the air fryer.
4) At 360° F or 183°C cook for 6 minutes. Cook in batches if required.

5) Serve and enjoy while eating.

Nutrition Information:

- Calories per Serving: 172
- Carbs: 4.8g
- Protein: 13.4g
- Fat: 10.9g

Sweet Honey-Hoisin Glazed Salmon

Servings per Recipe: 2

Cooking Time: 12 minutes

Ingredients:

- 1 tablespoon honey /15ML
- 1 tablespoon olive oil /15ML
- 1 tablespoon rice wine /15ML
- 1 tablespoon soy sauce /15ML
- 1-lb salmon filet, cut into 2-inch rectangles /450G
- 3 tablespoons hoisin sauce /45ML

Instructions:

1) Add all ingredients to a shallow bowl and mix properly. Allow to marinate in the refrigerator for 3 hours.
2) Thread salmon pieces in skewers and reserve marinade for sprinkling. Place on skewer rack in the air fryer.
3) At 360° F or 183°C cook for 12 minutes. Halfway through cooking time, turnover skewers and baste with marinade. If needed, cook in batches.
4) Serve and enjoy.

Nutrition Information:

- Calories per Serving: 971
- Carbs: 23.0g

- Protein: 139.4g
- Fat: 35.7g

Sweet-Chili Sauce Dip 'n Shrimp Rolls

Servings per Recipe: 8

Cooking Time: 9 minutes

Ingredients:

- ¼ teaspoon crushed red pepper /1.25G
- ½ cup sweet chili sauce /125ML
- ¾ cup snow peas, julienned /88G
- 1 cup carrots, julienned /130G
- 1 cup red bell pepper, seeded and julienned /130G
- 2 ½ tablespoons sesame oil, divided /38ML
- 2 cups cabbage, shredded /260G
- 2 teaspoons fish sauce /10ML
- 4 ounces raw shrimps, deveined and chopped /120G
- 8 spring roll wrappers

Instructions:

1) Place a saucepan over medium heat. Add sesame oil, add the cabbage, carrots, and bell pepper and stir for just two minutes. Set aside.
2) Once cooled, Add shrimps and snow peas. Season with fish sauce and red pepper.

3) Place the spring roll wrapper on a flat surface and put a
   tablespoon or two of the vegetable mixtures in the
   middle. Wrap the spring roll wrapper and seal the edges
   with water.
4) Preheat the air fryer to 390° F or 199°C.
5) Place the spring rolls in the double layer rack. Spray with
   olive oil.
6) Cook for 7 minutes.
7) Serve with chili sauce.

Nutrition information:

- Calories per serving: 185
- Carbs: 19g
- Protein: 7g
- Fat: 9g

Tartar Sauce 'n Crispy Cod Nuggets

Servings per Recipe: 3

Cooking Time: 10 Minutes

Ingredients:

- ½ cup flour /65G
- ½ cup non-fat mayonnaise /125ML
- ½ teaspoon Worcestershire sauce /2.5ML
- 1 ½ pounds cod fillet /675G
- 1 cup cracker crumbs /130G
- 1 egg, beaten
- 1 tablespoon sweet pickle relish /15G
- 1 tablespoon vegetable oil /15ML
- 1 teaspoon honey /5ML
- Juice from half a lemon
- Salt and pepper to taste
- Zest from half of a lemon

Instructions:

1) Preheat mid-air fryer to 390° F or 199°C .
2) Season the cod fillets with salt and pepper to taste.
3) Dip the fish in the flour, then in the beaten egg and then coat with the cracker crumbs. Brush all sides with oil.
4) Place the fish 'on the double layer rack and cook for 10 minutes.

5) Meanwhile, prepare the sauce by mixing all ingredients in
   a bowl.

6) Serve the fish using the sauce.

Nutrition information:

- Calories per serving: 470
- Carbs: 25.4g
- Protein: 42.9g
- Fat: 21.8g

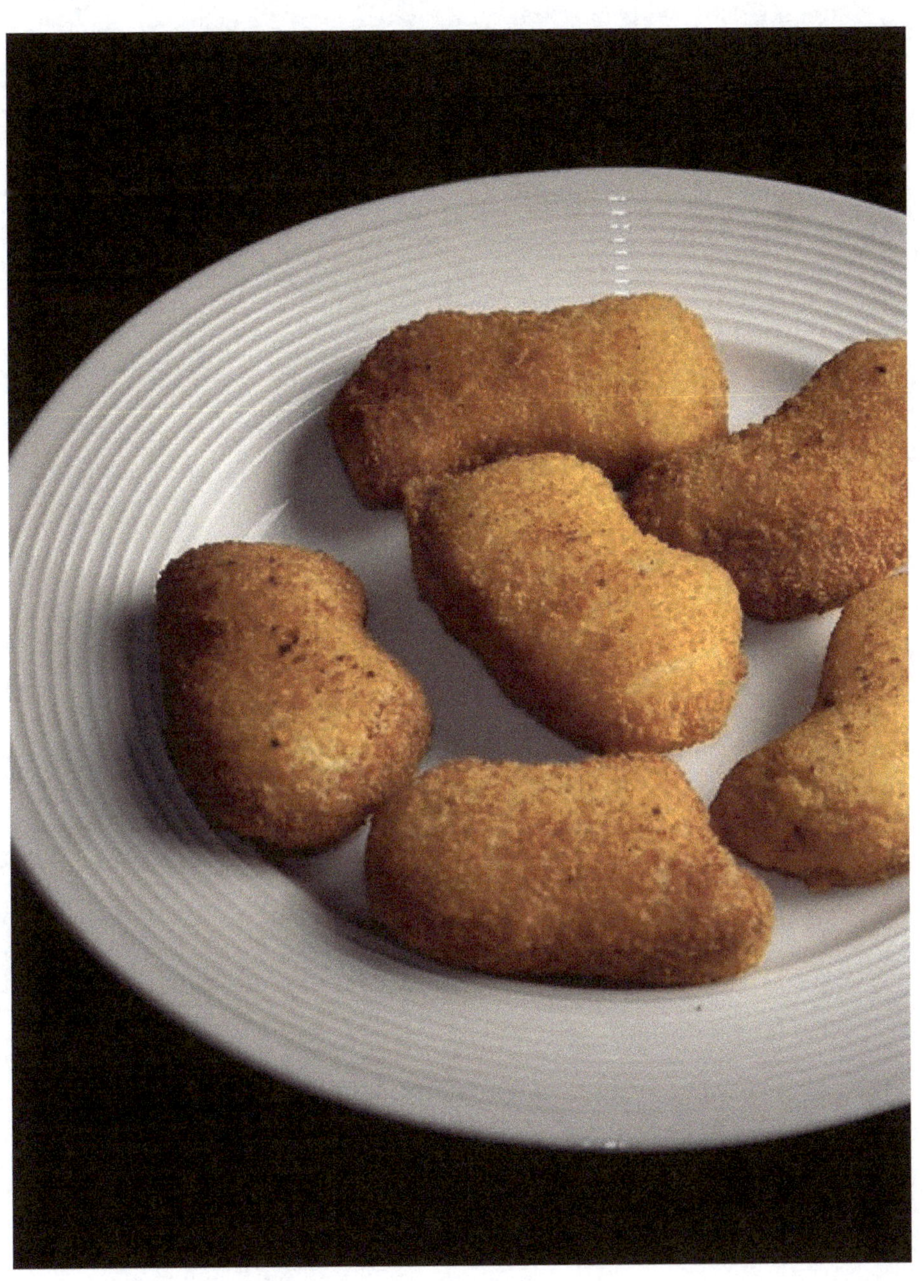

Tomato 'n Onion Stuffed Grilled Squid

Servings per Recipe: 4

Cooking Time: 15

Ingredients:

- ½ cup green onions, chopped /65G
- ½ cup tomatoes, chopped /65G
- 1 tablespoon fresh lemon juice /15ML
- 2 pounds squid, gutted and cleaned /900G
- 2 tablespoons organic olive oil /30ML
- 5 cloves of garlic
- Salt and pepper to taste

Instructions:

1) Preheat mid-air fryer to 390° F or 199°C .
2) Place the grill pan in the air fryer.
3) Season the squid with salt, pepper, and freshly squeezed lemon juice.
4) Stuff the hollow with garlic, tomatoes, and onions.
5) Brush the squid with essential olive oil.
6) Place on the grill pan and cook for 15 minutes.
7) Halfway through the cooking time, flip the squid.

Nutrition information:

- Calories per serving: 277

- Carbs: 10.7g
- Protein: 36g
- Fat: 10g

Tortilla-Crusted with Lemon Filets

Servings per Recipe: 4

Cooking Time: 15

Ingredients:

- 1 cup tortilla chips, pulverized /130G
- 1 egg, beaten
- 1 tablespoon lemon juice /15ML
- 4 fillets of white fish fillet
- Salt and pepper to taste

Instructions:

1) Preheat the air fryer to 390° F or 199°C .
2) Place a grill pan in the mid-air fryer.
3) Season the fish fillet with salt, pepper, and fresh lemon juice.
4) Drench in beaten eggs and also in tortilla chips.
5) Place in the grill pan.
6) Cook for 15. Minutes
7) Flip the fish halfway through the cooking time.

Nutrition information:

- Calories per serving: 300
- Carbs: 8.4g
- Protein: 24.8g

* Fat:18.6 g

Turmeric Spiced Salmon with Soy Sauce

Servings per Recipe: 4

Cooking Time: 12 minutes

Ingredients:

- ½ tablespoon sugar /7.5G
- ½ tablespoon turmeric powder /7.5G
- 1 cup cherry tomatoes /130G
- 1 slab of salmon fillets, sliced into cubes
- 1 tablespoon soy sauce /15ML
- A dash of black pepper
- Chopped coriander for garnish

Instructions:

1) Spice the salmon fillets with turmeric powder, sugar, soy sauce, and black pepper. Allow to marinate for 30 Minutes in the fridge.
2) Preheat air fryer to 330° F or 166°C .
3) Alternatively skewer the salmon cubes with tomatoes
4) Place on the double layer rack.
5) Cook for 10 to 12 minutes.

Nutrition information:

- Calories per serving: 302.3
- Carbs: 4.2g

- Protein: 47.3g
- Fat: 10.7g

Very Easy Lime-Garlic Shrimps

Servings per Recipe: 1

Cooking Time: 6 minutes

Ingredients:

- 1 clove of garlic, minced
- 1 cup raw shrimps /130G
- 1 lime, juiced and zested
- Salt and pepper to taste

Instructions:

1) Combine all ingredients in a mixing bowl and stir properly.
2) Preheat mid-air fryer to 390 O F or 199°C .
3) Wind the shrimps onto the steel skewers.
4) Place on the skewer rack and cook for 6 minutes.

Nutrition information:

- Calories per serving: 280
- Carbs: 8g
- Protein: 26g
- Fat: 16g

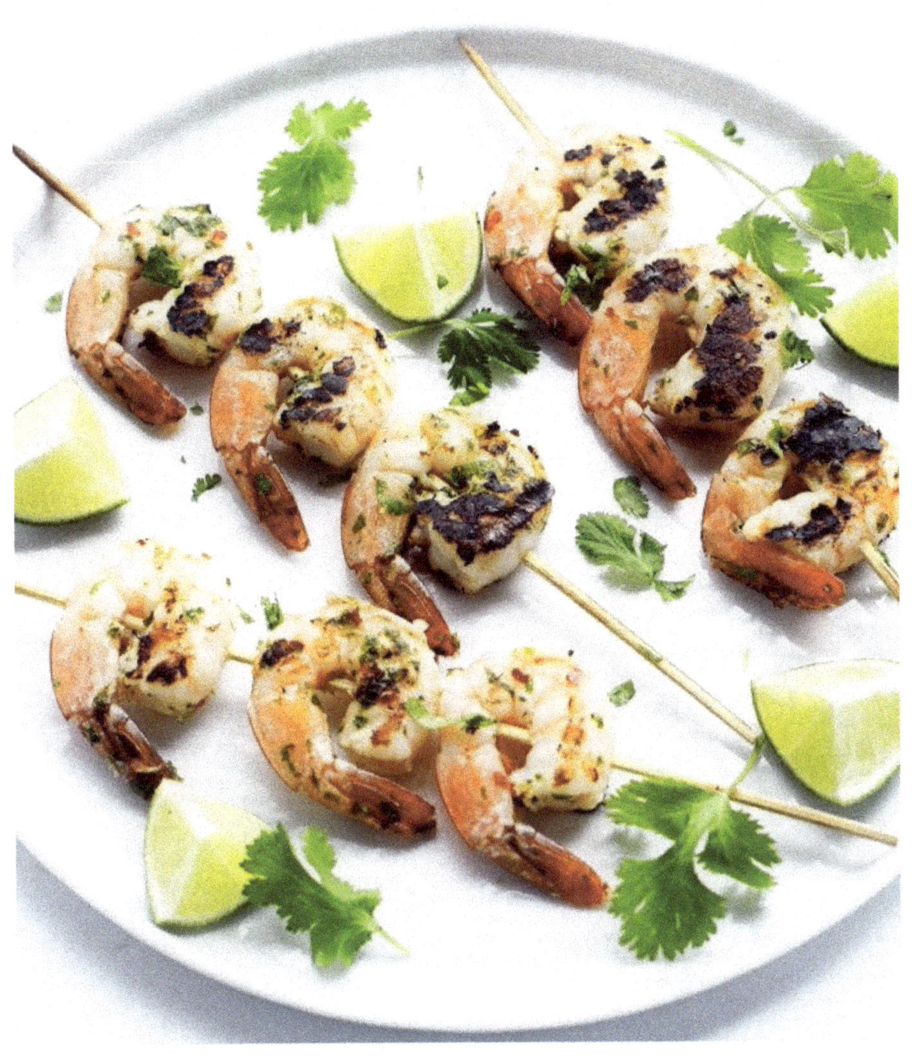

VEGETARIAN RECIPES

Almond Flour Battered 'n Crisped Onion Rings

Serves: 3

Cooking Time: 15 minutes

Ingredients:

- ½ cup almond flour /65G
- ¾ cup coconut milk /188ML
- 1 big white onion, sliced into rings
- 1 egg, beaten
- 1 tablespoon baking powder /15G
- 1 tablespoon smoked paprika /15G
- Salt and pepper to taste

Instructions:

1) Put on your air fryer and preheat for 5 minutes.
2) Add almond flour, baking powder, smoked paprika, salt and pepper in a mixing bowl. Mix properly until well combined.
3) Add eggs and coconut milk to another mixing bowl. Stir well to combine.
4) Dip the onion slices in the egg mixture.
5) Dip the onion slices again in the almond flour mixture.
6) Place in the air fryer basket and allow to cook at 325° F or 163°C for 15 minutes.

7) Shake the air fryer's basket halfway through cooking time.

Nutrition information:

- Calories per serving: 217
- Carbohydrates: 8.6g
- Protein: 5.3g
- Fat: 17.9g

Almond Flour Battered Wings

Serves: 4

Cooking Time: 25 minutes

Ingredients:

- ¼ cup butter, melted /32.5ML
- ¾ cup almond flour /98G
- 16 pieces of chicken wings
- 2 tablespoons stevia powder /30G
- 4 tablespoons minced garlic /60G
- Salt and pepper to taste

Instructions:

1) Put on your air fryer and preheat mid-air fryer for 5 minutes.
2) Add chicken wings, almond flour, stevia powder, and garlic in a mixing bowl. Add some salt and pepper to taste.
3) Put the seasoned chicken in an air fryer basket and cook for 25 minutes at 400° F or 205°C .
4) Shake the air fryer's basket halfway through the cooking time to ensure even doneness.
5) When done, remove the chicken, place it in a bowl and sprinkle it with melted butter. Flip severally to coat.

Nutrition information:

- Calories per serving: 365
- Carbohydrates: 7.8g
- Protein: 23.7g
- Fat: 26.9g

Baby Corn in Chili-Turmeric Spice

Serves: 5

Cooking Time: 8 minutes

Ingredients:

- ¼ cup water /62.5ML
- ¼ teaspoon baking soda /1.25G
- ¼ teaspoon salt /1.25G
- ¼ teaspoon turmeric powder /1.25G
- ½ teaspoon curry powder /2.5G
- ½ teaspoon red chili powder /2.5G
- 1 cup chickpea flour or besan /130G
- 10 pieces of baby corn, blanched

Instructions:

1) Put on your mid-air fryer and let it preheat to 400° F or 205°C .
2) Line the bottom of the air fryer basket with aluminium foil and lightly brush with any oil of your choice.
3) Mix all the above ingredients except the corn in a mixing bowl.
4) Whisk until well combined.
5) Coat the corn in the batter and place inside the air fryer. Cook for 8 minutes until golden brown.

Nutrition information:

- Calories per serving: 89
- Carbohydrates: 14.35g
- Protein: 4.75g
- Fat: 1.54g

Baked Cheesy Eggplant with Marinara

Servings per Recipe: 3

Cooking Time: 45 minutes

Ingredients:

- 1 clove garlic, sliced
- 1 large eggplants
- 1 tablespoon essential olive oil /15ML
- 1 tablespoon organic olive oil /15ML
- 1/2 pinch salt, or as required
- 1/4 cup and 2 tablespoons dry bread crumbs /62.5G
- 1/4 cup and a pair of tablespoons ricotta cheese /62.5G
- 1/4 cup grated Parmesan cheese /32.5G
- 1/4 cup grated Parmesan cheese /32.5G
- 1/4 cup water, and many more as required /62.5
- 1/4 teaspoon red pepper flakes /1.25G
- 1-1/2 cups prepared marinara sauce /375ML
- 1-1/2 teaspoons extra virgin olive oil /7.5ML
- 2 tablespoons shredded pepper jack cheese /10G
- salt and freshly ground black pepper to taste

Instructions:

1. Chop the eggplant diagonally into 5 pieces. Peel off the rind and chop two pieces into ½-inch cubes.

2. Sprinkle the baking pan of the air fryer with 1 tbsp or 15 ML olive oil. Heat the oil at 390° F or 199°C for 5 minutes. Add half the chopped eggplant and cook for two main minutes per side. Set in a plate.

3. Add 1 ½ tsp extra virgin olive oil and add garlic. Cook for a minute. Add chopped eggplants. Season with pepper flakes and salt. Cook for 4 minutes. Lower heat to 330° F or 166°C and continue cooking eggplants until soft, for about 8 more minutes.

4. While stirring add water and marinara sauce. Cook for 7 minutes until heated through. Stirring from time to time. Transfer to a bowl.

5. In a bowl, whisk well pepper, salt, pepper jack cheese, Parmesan cheese, and ricotta. Evenly spread cheeses over eggplant strips then fold in two.

6. Lay folded eggplant in baking pan. Pour the marinara sauce on the top.

7. In a small bowl whisk well organic olive oil, and bread crumbs. Sprinkle all over the sauce.

8. Cook for 15 at 390°F or 199°C until tops are lightly browned.

9. Serve and get.

Nutrition Information:

- Calories per Serving: 405
- Carbs: 41.1g

- Protein: 12.7g
- Fat: 21.4g

Baked Polenta with Chili-Cheese

Servings per Recipe: 3

Cooking Time: 10 Minutes

Ingredients:

- 1 commercial polenta roll, sliced
- 1 cup cheddar cheese sauce /130G
- 1 tablespoon chili powder /15G

Instructions:

1) To start the preparation of this meal first put the baking pan in mid-air fryer.
2) Then arrange the polenta slices in the baking pan.
3) Add the chili powder and cheddar cheese sauce to the slices.
4) Close mid-air fryer and cook for 10 minutes at 390° F or 199°C .

Nutrition information:

- Calories per serving: 206
- Carbs: 25.3g
- Protein: 3.2g
- Fat: 4.2g

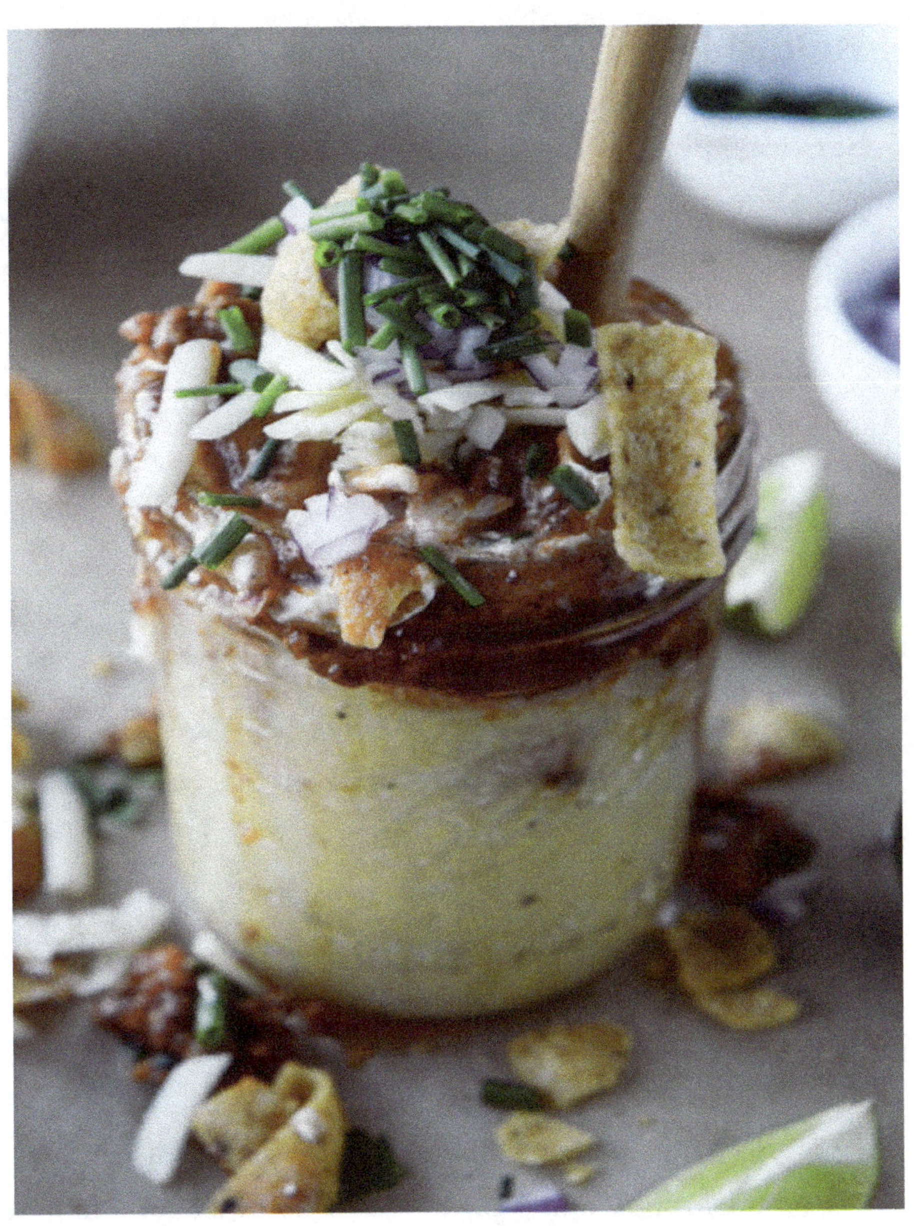

Baked Portobello, Pasta 'n Cheese

Servings per Recipe: 4

Cooking Time: 30 Minutes

Ingredients:

- 1 cup milk /250ML
- 1 cup shredded mozzarella cheese /130G
- 1 large clove garlic, minced
- 1 tablespoon vegetable oil /15ML
- 1/4 cup margarine /32.5G
- 1/4 teaspoon dried basil /32.5G
- 1/4-pound portobello mushrooms, thinly sliced /112.5G
- 2 tablespoons all-purpose flour /30G
- 2 tablespoons soy sauce /30ML
- 4-ounce penne pasta, cooked according to manufacturer's Directions for Cooking /120G
- 5-ounce frozen chopped spinach, thawed /150G

Instructions:

1) Spray the Baking pan lightly with oil to grease it. Add mushrooms and cook at 360 ° F or 183°C for 2 minutes, when done place on a plate.

2) Add margarine to the same baking pan, allow to melt for a minute. Add the basil, garlic, and flour. Stir. Allow cooking for 3 minutes. While stirring add 50 % of the milk slowly. Stir continuously. Allow cooking for the next 2 minutes. Mix well. Add the remaining milk while still stirring and allow to cook for additional 3 more minutes.

3) Add the cheese and stir well.

4) Add the soy sauce, spinach, mushrooms, and pasta. Mix well. Add the remaining cheese.

5) Cook for 15 minutes at 390° F or 199°C until toppings are lightly browned.

6) Serve and enjoy.

Nutrition Information:

- Calories per Serving: 482
- Carbs: 32.1g
- Protein: 16.0g
- Fat: 32.1g

Baked Potato Topped with Cream cheese 'n Olives

Serves: 1

Cooking Time: 40 minutes

Ingredients:

- ¼ teaspoon onion powder /1.25G
- 1 medium russet potato, scrubbed and peeled
- 1 tablespoon chives, chopped /15G
- 1 tablespoon Kalamata olives /15G
- 1 teaspoon essential olive oil /5ML
- 1/8 teaspoon salt /0.625G
- a dollop of vegan butter
- a dollop of vegan cream cheese

Instructions:

1) Preheat the air fryer to 400° F or 205°C
2) Place the potatoes inside a mixing bowl and add extra virgin olive oil, onion powder, salt, and vegan butter.
3) Place inside the air fryer basket and cook for 40 minutes. Be sure to turn the potatoes once halfway through cooking time
4) Serve the potatoes with vegan cream cheese, Kalamata olives, chives, as well as other vegan toppings that you want.

Nutrition information:

- Calories per serving: 504
- Carbohydrates: 68.34g
- Protein: 9.31g
- Fat: 21.53g

Baked Zucchini Recipe From Mexico

Servings per Recipe: 4

Cooking Time: 30 minutes

Ingredients:

- 1 tablespoon olive oil /15ML
- 1-1/2 pounds zucchini, cubed /675G
- 1/2 cup chopped onion /65G
- 1/2 teaspoon garlic salt /2.5G
- 1/2 teaspoon paprika /2.5G
- 1/2 teaspoon dried oregano /2.5G
- 1/2 teaspoon cayenne pepper, or to taste /2.5G
- 1/2 cup cooked long-grain rice /65G
- 1/2 cup cooked pinto beans /65G
- 1-1/4 cups salsa /195G
- 3/4 cup shredded Cheddar cheese /88G

Instructions:

1) Spray the baking pan lightly with any oil of your choice to grease it. Drop in onions and zucchini in the pan and allow to cook for 10 minutes at 360O F or 183°C .
2) Add cayenne, oregano, paprika, garlic salt and stir.
3) While stirring add salsa, beans, and rice. Cook for 5 minutes.
4) Also add cheddar cheese and stir well.

5) Cover the pan with aluminium foil.

6) Let it cook for 15 minutes at 390 **O** F or 199°C .

7) Serve and enjoy.

Nutrition Information:

- Calories per Serving: 263
- Carbs: 24.6g
- Protein: 12.5g
- Fat: 12.7g

Banana Pepper Stuffed with Tofu 'n Spices

Serves: 8

Cooking Time: 10 minutes

Ingredients:

- ½ teaspoon red chili powder /2.5G
- ½ teaspoon turmeric powder /2.5G
- 1 onion, finely chopped
- 1 package firm tofu, crumbled
- 1 teaspoon coriander powder /5G
- 3 tablespoons coconut oil /15ML
- 8 banana peppers, top quality sliced and seeded
- Salt to taste

Instructions:

1) Allow mid-air fryer to warm up for 5 minutes.
2) Add the tofu, onion, coconut oil, turmeric powder, red chili powder, coriander powder, and salt to a mixing bowl. Stir well until properly combined.
3) Using a spoon take a portion of the tofu mixture and place it in the holes of the banana peppers.
4) Place the stuffed peppers in the air fryer.
5) Allow cooking for 10 Minutes at 325° F or 163°C .

Nutrition information:

- Calories per serving: 72
- Carbohydrates: 4.1g
- Protein: 1.2g
- Fat: 5.6g

Bell Pepper-Corn Wrapped in Tortilla

Serves: 4

Cooking Time: 15

Ingredients:

- 1 small red bell pepper, chopped
- 1 small yellow onion, diced
- 1 tablespoon water /15ML
- 2 cobs grilled corn kernels
- 4 large tortillas
- 4 pieces commercial vegan nuggets, chopped
- mixed greens for garnish

Instructions:

1) Warm up the air fryer to 400° F or 205°C .
2) Sauté the onions, bell peppers, and corn kernels using water over medium heat in a pan. Set aside.
3) Place filling inside corn tortillas.
4) Fold the tortillas and put them inside a mid-air fryer and cook for 15 minutes before the tortilla wraps are crispy.
5) Serve with mixed greens ahead.

Nutrition information:

- Calories per serving: 548
- Carbohydrates: 43.54g

- Protein: 46.73g
- Fat: 20.76g

Black Bean Burger with Garlic-Chipotle

Servings per Recipe: 3

Cooking Time: 20 minutes

Ingredients:

- ½ cup corn kernels /65G
- ½ teaspoon chipotle powder /2.5G
- ½ teaspoon garlic powder /2.5G
- ¾ cup salsa /88G
- 1 ¼ teaspoon chili powder /6.25G
- 1 ½ cup rolled oats /195G
- 1 can black beans, rinsed and drained
- 1 tablespoon soy sauce /15ML

Instructions:

1) Add all ingredients to a mixing bowl and mix using your hands.
2) Make small lumps of the constituent with your hands and hang upside down.
3) Polish the pastry lump with oil (Optional).
4) Place the grill pan in the air fryer and place the pastry lump in the pan.
5) Cook for 20 minutes on both sides at 330° F or 166°C . Ensure both sides are evenly brown.

Nutrition information:

- Calories per serving: 395

- Carbs: 52.2g

- Protein: 24.3g

- Fat: 5.8g

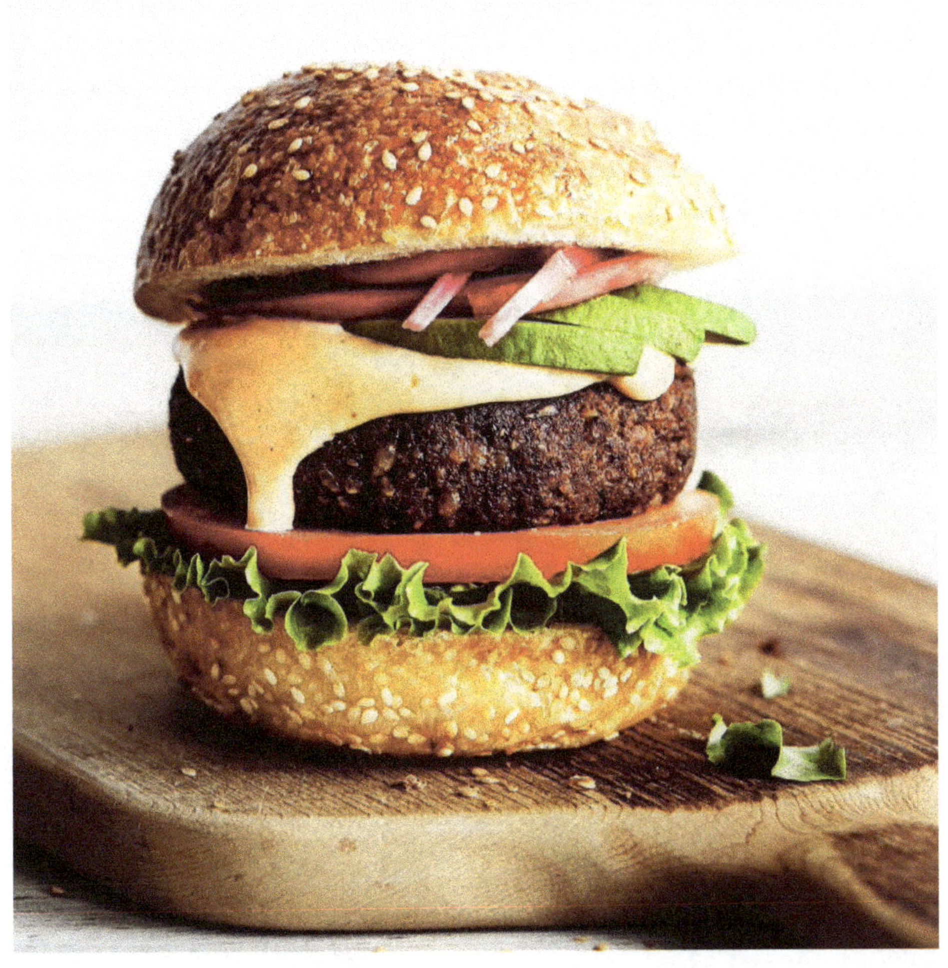

CPSIA information can be obtained
at www.ICGtesting.com
Printed in the USA
LVHW080817300721
693916LV00002B/105